PLANT BASED KIDNEY STONE COOKBOOK

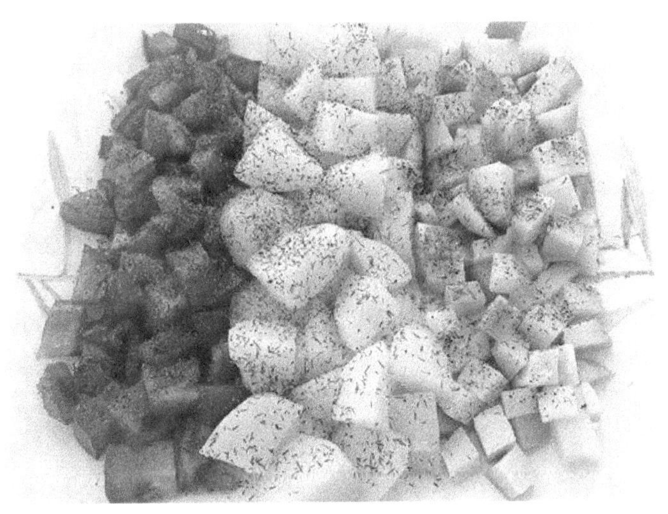

Dr. Mary Dixon

Copyright © 2023 by Dr. Mary Dixon

All rights reserved. No part of this publication may be reproduced, distributed, or transmitted in any form or by any means, including photocopying, recording, or other electronic or mechanical methods, without the prior written permission of the publisher, except in the case of brief quotations embodied in critical reviews and certain other noncommercial uses permitted by copyright law.

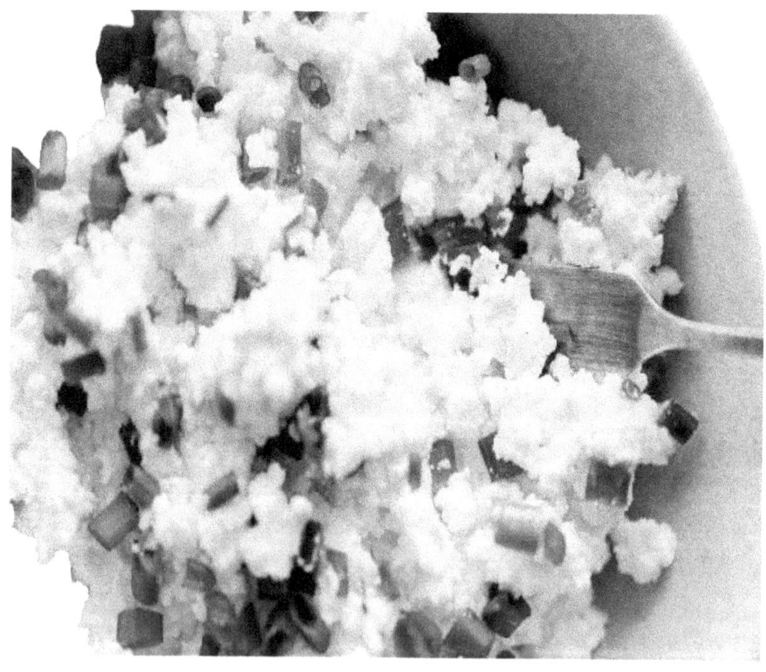

Table of Contents

INTRODUCTION

Emily had been suffering from chronic kidney stones for years. She had tried everything - medication, surgery, and even alternative therapies like acupuncture, but nothing seemed to work. The pain was unbearable, and she was tired of feeling helpless.

One day, Emily's friend suggested that she try a plant-based diet to cure her kidney stones. At first, Emily was sceptical. How could something as simple as changing her diet make a difference? But she had to try since she was so eager for relief.

Emily started by cutting out all animal products and processed foods from her diet. She replaced them with whole, plant-based foods like fruits, vegetables, legumes, and whole grains. To stay hydrated, she also made sure to drink a lot of water.

At first, Emily didn't notice any changes. But after a few weeks, she started to feel better. Her energy levels improved, and the pain in her kidneys began to subside.

She couldn't believe it - after years of suffering, a simple change in diet had made all the difference.

Emily continued with her plant-based diet, and over time, her kidney stones disappeared completely. She was amazed by how much her diet had affected her health and vowed to never go back to her old eating habits.

As Emily looked back on her journey, she realized that sometimes the simplest solutions can be the most effective. She was grateful for her friend's suggestion and for the healing power of plants.

Emily's story inspired others to make positive changes in their diets, and she was happy to share her newfound knowledge with others who were struggling with health issues like hers.

Kidney stones, also known as renal calculi, are small, solid deposits that form in the kidneys from waste products in the urine.

These stones can range in size from a grain of sand to a golf ball, and can cause intense pain and discomfort as they travel through the urinary tract.

The kidneys are responsible for filtering waste products from the blood and producing urine, which is then passed through the urinary tract and out of the body. However, sometimes these waste products can become concentrated and form crystals, which then join together to form kidney stones.

Kidney stones are a common condition, affecting approximately 1 in 10 people at some point in their lives.

They are more common in men than women, and can occur at any age, although they are more commonly seen in adults aged 30-60 years.

Risk factors for developing kidney stones include a family history of the condition, dehydration, obesity, and certain medical conditions such as gout or inflammatory bowel disease.

Symptoms of kidney stones can vary depending on the size and location of the stone, but can include severe pain in the back or side, nausea and vomiting, fever, and pain or burning during urination.

In some cases, kidney stones can also cause blood in the urine, or frequent urination.

The type of treatment for kidney stones depends on the size, location, and intensity of the symptoms. Smaller stones may pass on their own through the urinary tract, while larger stones may require medical intervention such as shock wave lithotripsy (using shock waves to break up) Surgery, ureteroscopy (using a tiny scope to remove the stone), or other methods can be used.

Prevention of kidney stones involves staying well hydrated, eating a balanced diet low in salt and animal protein, and avoiding certain foods that can increase the risk of stone formation, such as spinach, rhubarb, and chocolate.

In some cases, medication may also be prescribed to prevent the formation of kidney stones.

Overall, while kidney stones can be a painful and uncomfortable condition, prompt diagnosis and treatment can help to manage symptoms and prevent complications.

CHAPTER ONE

Plant Based Kidney Stone Explained

There are millions of people who experience kidney stones worldwide. They occur when small, hard deposits of mineral and acid salts form in the kidneys, which can cause excruciating pain when they pass through the urinary tract.

While there are many different types of kidney stones, some research suggests that a plant-based diet may be helpful in reducing the risk of certain types of kidney stones.

Plant-based diets, which focus on eating whole, unprocessed foods such as fruits, vegetables, whole grains, legumes, and nuts, have been shown to have numerous health benefits.

They are associated with lower rates of heart disease, diabetes, and certain types of cancer, as well as improved overall health and longevity.

In addition to these benefits, some studies suggest that a plant-based diet may also help prevent the formation of kidney stones.

One reason why plant-based diets may be helpful in preventing kidney stones is because they tend to be lower in animal protein.

Animal protein, particularly from red meat and poultry, is associated with an increased risk of developing kidney stones.

When the body digests animal protein, it produces more acid, which can increase the level of calcium in the urine. This, in turn, can lead to the formation of calcium oxalate stones, which are the most common type of kidney stone.

In contrast, plant-based diets tend to be higher in fibre, which can help reduce the absorption of calcium and other minerals in the intestines. This, in turn, can help lower the amount of calcium in the urine and reduce the risk of developing kidney stones.

Additionally, plant-based diets tend to be rich in a variety of nutrients, including magnesium and potassium, which have been shown to be helpful in preventing kidney stones.

One study that looked at the effect of a plant-based diet on kidney stone risk found that people who followed a vegetarian or vegan diet had a lower risk of developing kidney stones compared to those who ate a diet that included meat. Another study found that people who followed a low-fat, vegan diet had a significantly lower risk of developing kidney stones compared to those who ate a standard American diet.

While more research is needed to fully understand the relationship between plant-based diets and kidney stones, the evidence suggests that a plant-based diet may be helpful in reducing the risk of certain types of kidney stones.

If you are concerned about your risk of developing kidney stones, it may be worth talking to your doctor or a registered dietitian about incorporating more plant-based foods into your diet.

By making simple changes like eating more fruits, vegetables, whole grains, legumes, and nuts, you may be able to reduce your risk of kidney stones and enjoy a range of other health benefits as well.

Types of Kidney Stone

Kidney stones, also known as renal calculi, are hard mineral deposits that form inside the kidneys and can cause severe pain when they move through the urinary tract.

The most common types of kidney stones are made up of calcium oxalate, but there are several other types that can also form.

Here are the types of kidney stones, along with a brief explanation of their composition and characteristics:

1. **Calcium Oxalate Stones:** These are the most common type of kidney stones, accounting for about 80% of all cases. They form when calcium and oxalate combine in the urine to create a crystal-like substance that can become trapped in the kidneys or urinary tract.

2. **Struvite Stones:** These stones are composed of magnesium, ammonium, and phosphate, and are often associated with urinary tract infections. They have a high rate of growth and can get fairly big.

3. **Uric Acid Stones:** These stones form when there is an excess of uric acid in the urine. They are more likely to form in people who have gout or who consume a high-protein diet.

4. **Cystine Stones:** These stones are rare and are caused by a genetic disorder that leads to an excess of cystine in the urine. They tend to be larger than other types of kidney stones and can cause severe pain.

5. **Calcium Phosphate Stones:** These stones are less common than calcium oxalate stones, but can still cause significant pain and discomfort. They form when calcium and phosphate combine in the urine to create a crystal-like substance that can become trapped in the kidneys or urinary tract.

It is important to note that the treatment for kidney stones can vary depending on the type of stone, so it is important to get an accurate diagnosis from a healthcare professional.

Causes of Kidney Stone

Kidney stones are solid, hard deposits that form in the kidneys or urinary tract when there is an imbalance of minerals, salts, and other substances in the urine. When going through the urinary tract, they can cause excruciating pain and agony.

There are several causes of kidney stones, which can be broadly categorized as follows:

1. **Dehydration:** When the body doesn't get enough water, the urine becomes concentrated, which can lead to the formation of kidney stones.

2. **Diet:** Kidney stone production is more likely in people who consume large amounts of salt, sugar, and animal protein. Consuming too much oxalate-rich foods like spinach, rhubarb, and chocolate can also lead to the formation of calcium oxalate stones.

3. **Genetics:** A family history of kidney stones increases the likelihood of developing them.

4. **Medical conditions:** Certain medical conditions like gout, inflammatory bowel disease, and urinary tract infections can increase the risk of kidney stone formation.

5. **Medications:** Some medications like diuretics, calcium-based antacids, and certain antibiotics can increase the risk of kidney stone formation.

6. **Obesity:** Kidney stones are more likely to form in overweight or obese people.

7. **Other factors:** Other factors like a sedentary lifestyle, excessive alcohol consumption, and certain surgical procedures can also increase the risk of kidney stone formation.

It's important to note that many people with risk factors for kidney stones never develop them, while others may develop them without any apparent risk factors. If you suspect you have a kidney stone, it's important to consult with a healthcare professional for proper diagnosis and treatment.

Symptoms of Kidney Stone

1. **Pain:** This is the most common symptom of kidney stones, and is often described as a sharp, intense pain that can come and go in waves. The pain is usually felt in the back, side, lower abdomen, or groin.

2. **Difficulty urinating:** Kidney stones can cause a blockage in the urinary tract, making it difficult or painful to urinate. Some people may feel a constant urge to urinate, even if they are unable to pass much urine.

3. **Blood in the urine:** Kidney stones can cause small amounts of blood to appear in the urine, which may be visible or only detected with a microscope.

4. **Nausea and vomiting:** Especially if the pain is intense, some kidney stone sufferers may feel nausea and vomiting.

5. **Fever and chills:** In some cases, kidney stones can cause an infection in the urinary tract, which may lead to fever and chills.

6. **Foul-smelling urine:** If an infection is present, the urine may have a strong, unpleasant odour.

7. **Cloudy or discoloured urine:** The presence of kidney stones can cause the urine to become cloudy or discoloured, which may indicate the presence of blood or infection.

Overall, the symptoms of kidney stones can vary depending on the size and location of the stone, as well as other factors such as the presence of infection or other medical conditions.

It's crucial to see a healthcare professional if you have any of these symptoms in order to have a precise diagnosis and the best course of action.

Kidney Stone Prevention

1. **Stay hydrated:** Drinking enough fluids is one of the most important things you can do to prevent kidney stones. If you are physically active or live in a hot area, aim for at least 8 to 10 glasses of water per day. Staying hydrated helps dilute the urine and prevents minerals from crystallizing and forming stones.

2. **Reduce sodium intake:** Excessive sodium intake can increase the risk of kidney stone formation. Limit your intake of processed and packaged foods, which tend to be high in sodium. Instead, opt for fresh fruits and vegetables, lean proteins, and whole grains.

3. **Limit animal protein:** Animal proteins, such as meat, fish, and poultry, can increase the concentration of calcium and uric acid in the urine, which can contribute to the formation of kidney stones. Consider reducing your intake of animal protein and opting for plant-based protein sources instead.

4. **Get enough calcium:** Contrary to common opinion, having a diet high in calcium can help prevent kidney stones. Calcium binds to oxalate in the intestine, preventing it from being absorbed into the bloodstream and excreted in the urine. Aim for 1,000-1,200 mg of calcium per day from food sources such as milk, cheese, and leafy greens.

5. **Limit oxalate-rich foods:** Oxalate is a compound found in many foods, including spinach, rhubarb, and chocolate, that can increase the risk of kidney stone formation. While it's important to eat a balanced diet that includes these foods, consider limiting your intake of them if you have a history of kidney stones.

6. **Talk to your doctor about medications:** Depending on your individual risk factors for kidney stones, your doctor may recommend medications to help prevent their formation. These may include thiazide diuretics, allopurinol, or potassium citrate.

By following these tips, you can reduce your risk of developing kidney stones and enjoy better urinary tract health.

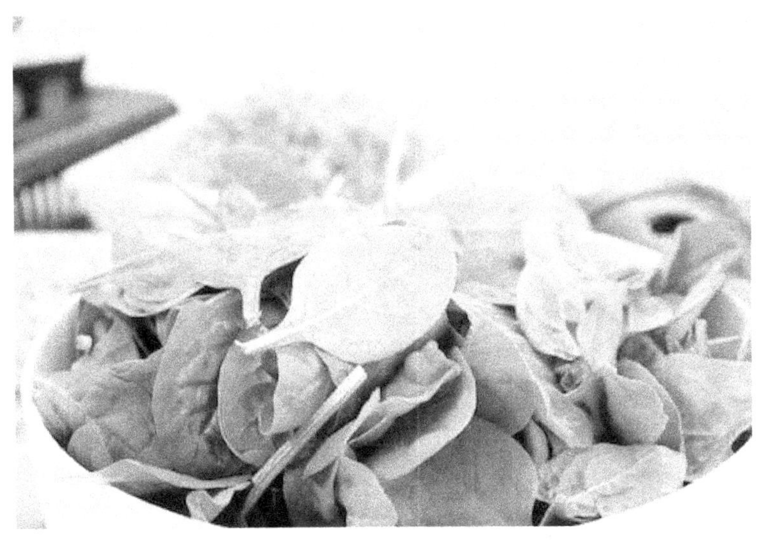

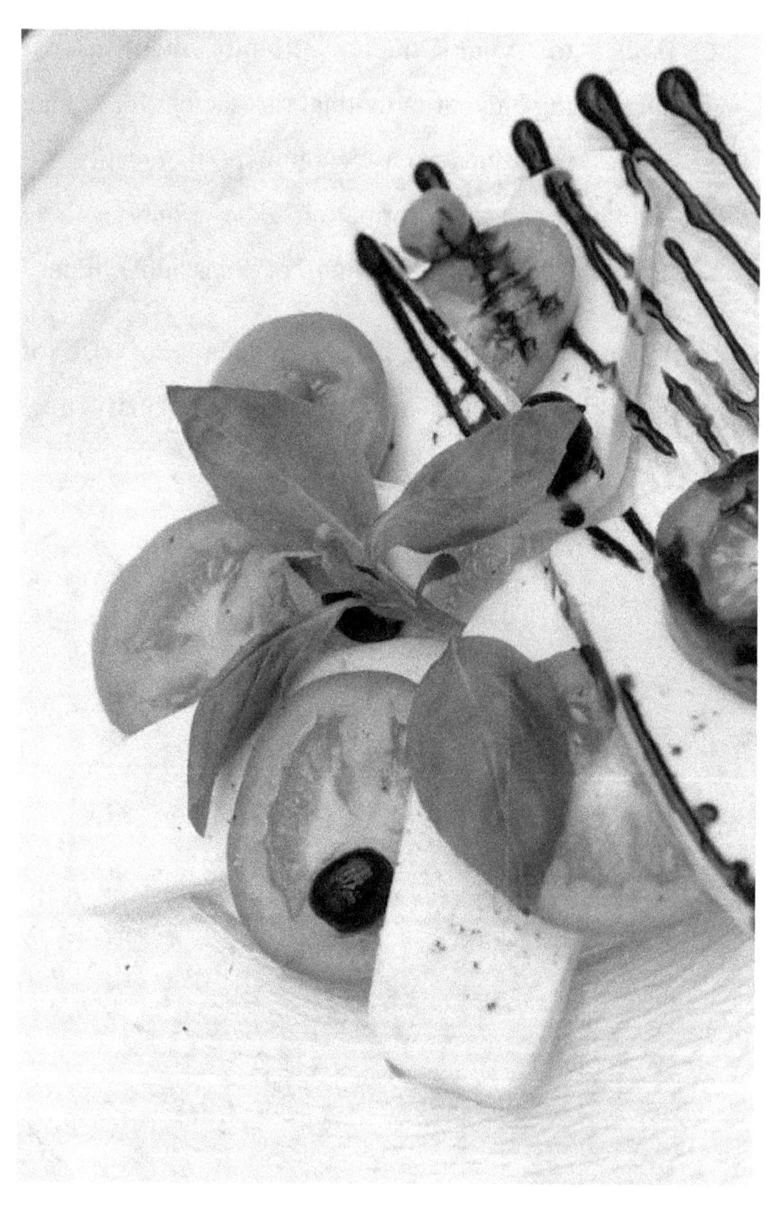

CHAPTER TWO

Kidney Stone Diet and Benefits

What is a kidney stone diet?

A kidney stone diet is a diet that is low in certain types of foods that can contribute to the formation of kidney stones. This includes foods that are high in oxalate, a substance that can bind with calcium in the urine and form kidney stones. Foods that are high in animal protein, sodium, and sugar can also increase the risk of kidney stones.The goal of a kidney stone diet is to reduce the amount of these substances in the body and promote a healthy balance of minerals in the urine. By doing so, the risk of kidney stone formation can be greatly reduced.

Benefits of a kidney stone Diet

Reduces the risk of kidney stones

As mentioned earlier, the primary benefit of a kidney stone diet is its ability to reduce the risk of kidney stone formation. By limiting the intake of foods that are high in oxalate, animal protein, sodium, and sugar, the body is less likely to form kidney stones.

Promotes overall health

A kidney stone diet is also beneficial for overall health. It encourages the consumption of fresh fruits and vegetables, which are rich in vitamins, minerals, and fibre. It also promotes a healthy weight, which can reduce the risk of other health problems such as heart disease and diabetes.

Can improve kidney function

A kidney stone diet can also improve kidney function. By reducing the workload on the kidneys and promoting a healthy balance of minerals in the urine, the kidneys are better able to function properly.

Tips for implementing a kidney stone Diet

Drink plenty of water

One of the most crucial things you can do to avoid kidney stones is to drink enough of water. Water helps to dilute the concentration of minerals in the urine, making it less likely that they will bind together and form stones. Aim to consume eight glasses of water or more each day.

Limit high-oxalate foods

Foods that are high in oxalate include spinach, rhubarb, beets, nuts, chocolate, and tea. While these foods are still healthy and can be consumed in moderation, it is important to limit their intake if you are at risk for kidney stones.

Reduce animal protein intake

Animal protein can increase the amount of calcium in the urine, which can contribute to kidney stone formation. Limit your intake of meat, poultry, and fish to no more than 6 ounces per day.

Cut back on sodium and sugar

Kidney stones can also be made more likely by sodium and sugar. Limit your intake of processed foods, which are often high in both of these substances. Choose fresh foods instead, and use herbs and spices to add flavour instead of salt.

In conclusion, a kidney stone diet can be an effective way to prevent kidney stones from forming. By limiting the intake of foods that are high in oxalate, animal protein, sodium, and sugar, the body is less likely to form stones. In addition to reducing the risk of kidney stones, a kidney stone diet can also promote overall health and improve kidney function. If you are at risk for kidney stones, talk to your doctor or a registered dietitian to develop a plan that works for you.

How to Follow a Plant Based Kidney Stone Diet

Kidney stones are a common condition affecting many people worldwide. They occur when small crystals form in the urine and combine to create a hard, rock-like substance. People who have experienced kidney stones know how painful and uncomfortable they can be, and it's important to take steps to prevent them from forming in the first place.

One of the ways to prevent kidney stones is by following a plant-based diet. Plant-based diets are rich in nutrients, fibre, and antioxidants, and they can help reduce the risk of kidney stones by promoting urinary excretion of calcium and oxalate, two substances that can contribute to stone formation.

In this book, we'll explore the benefits of a plant-based kidney stone diet and provide some tips and recommendations for following one.

Benefits of a Plant-Based Kidney Stone Diet:

1. **High in Fibre:** Plant-based diets are typically high in fibre, which can help regulate bowel movements and prevent constipation. This is important because constipation can lead to the build-up of waste products in the body, which can contribute to the formation of kidney stones.

2. **Rich in Nutrients:** Plant-based diets are rich in essential nutrients such as vitamins, minerals, and antioxidants. These nutrients can help support overall health and well-being, as well as promote the excretion of calcium and oxalate in the urine.

3. **Low in Sodium:** Plant-based diets are typically low in sodium, which is important because high levels of sodium can contribute to the formation of kidney stones. Reducing sodium intake can also help lower blood pressure and improve overall heart health.

Tips for Following a Plant-Based Kidney Stone Diet:

1. **Increase Intake of Fruits and Vegetables:** Fruits and vegetables are an essential part of a plant-based diet, and they are rich in essential nutrients and fibre. Incorporate a range of vibrant fruits and vegetables into your diet on a daily basis.

2. **Choose Whole Grains:** Whole grains are an excellent source of fibre and nutrients, and they can help regulate blood sugar levels and reduce the risk of heart disease. Instead of refined carbohydrates like white rice and white bread, choose whole grains like brown rice, quinoa, and whole wheat bread.

3. **Limit Animal Protein:** Animal protein can contribute to the formation of kidney stones, so it's important to limit your intake of meat, poultry, and fish. Instead, opt for plant-based sources of protein like beans, lentils, and tofu.

4. **Drink Plenty of Water:** Staying hydrated is essential for preventing kidney stones.

Aim to consume eight glasses of water a day or more if you exercise frequently or live in a warm region.

5. **Avoid High-Oxalate Foods:** Some plant-based foods are high in oxalate, which can contribute to the formation of kidney stones. Foods to avoid or limit include spinach, rhubarb, beets, nuts, and chocolate.

6. **Use Lemon Juice:** Lemon juice is a natural source of citrate, which can help prevent the formation of kidney stones. Try adding a squeeze of lemon juice to your water or using it as a salad dressing.

Following a plant-based kidney stone diet can be a delicious and nutritious way to prevent kidney stones.

By increasing your intake of fruits and vegetables, choosing whole grains, limiting animal protein, staying hydrated, avoiding high-oxalate foods, and using lemon juice, you can reduce your risk of kidney stone formation and promote overall health and well-being. Don't forget to talk to your doctor before making any big dietary adjustments.

7 Day Plant Based Kidney Stone Meal Plan

Day 1

Breakfast:

Overnight Oats with Blueberries and Almonds

Ingredients:

- 1/2 cup rolled oats

- 1/2 cup almond milk

- 1/2 cup fresh blueberries

- 1 tbsp chopped almonds

Preparation Method:

1. In a bowl, combine oats and almond milk. Stir well.

2. Add blueberries and stir gently.

3. Place the bowl in the refrigerator overnight with the lid on.

4. In the morning, top with chopped almonds and serve.

Lunch:

Grilled Vegetable Salad

Ingredients:

- 1 zucchini, sliced lengthwise

- 1 yellow squash, sliced lengthwise

- 1 red bell pepper, sliced

- 1 tbsp olive oil

- 2 cups mixed greens

- 1/4 cup walnuts

- 2 tbsp balsamic vinegar

- Salt and pepper, to taste

Preparation Method:

1. Preheat grill to medium-high heat.

2. Olive oil should be used to brush vegetables before adding salt and pepper.

3. Grill vegetables for 2-3 minutes on each side, until lightly charred and tender.

4. Arrange mixed greens on a plate and top with grilled vegetables and walnuts.

5. Drizzle balsamic vinegar over the salad and serve.

Dinner:

Lentil and Vegetable Stir Fry

Ingredients:

- 1 cup cooked lentils

- 1 cup mixed vegetables (carrots, broccoli, cauliflower, and bell peppers)

- 1 tbsp olive oil

- 1 clove garlic, minced

- 1 tbsp low-sodium soy sauce

- 1/4 tsp red pepper flakes

Preparation Method:

1. Olive oil should be heated in a big pan over a medium-high heat.

2. Add garlic and stir for 1 minute.

3. Mixture of vegetables should be stir-fried for two to three minutes, or until soft.

4. Add cooked lentils, soy sauce, and red pepper flakes. Stir well.

5. Cook for a further 1-2 minutes, or until well cooked.

6. Serve hot.

Day 2

Breakfast:

Spinach and Mushroom Omelette

Ingredients:

- 2 eggs

- 1/2 cup chopped spinach

- 1/4 cup sliced mushrooms

- 1 tbsp olive oil

- Salt and pepper, to taste

Preparation Method:

1. Beat the eggs with salt and pepper in a bowl.

2. Olive oil should be heated over medium heat in a non-stick pan.

3. Add chopped spinach and sliced mushrooms to the pan. Cook for 2-3 minutes, until tender.

4. Pour the beaten eggs into the pan.

5. Use a spatula to lift the edges of the omelette and allow the uncooked eggs to flow underneath.

6. Once the omelette is cooked through, fold it in half and serve.

Lunch:

Tomato and Avocado Sandwich

Ingredients:

- 2 slices of whole-grain bread

- 1 small avocado, sliced

- 1 medium tomato, sliced

- 1 tbsp hummus

- Salt and pepper, to taste

Preparation Method:

1. Toast the bread slices.

2. On one side of each slice of bread, spread hummus.

3. Top one slice of bread with avocado slices, and the other slice with tomato slices.

4. Season with salt and pepper.

5. Place the avocado and tomato slices together to form a sandwich.

6. Cut in half and serve.

Dinner:

Black Bean and Sweet Potato Enchiladas

Ingredients:

- 6 whole-grain tortillas

- 1 can black beans, drained and rinsed

- 1 medium sweet potato, peeled and diced

- 1/2 onion, diced

- 2 garlic cloves, minced

- 1 tsp cumin

- 1 tsp chili powder

- 1 cup vegetable broth

- 1 cup salsa

- 1 cup shredded vegan cheese

- Salt and pepper, to taste

Preparation Method:

1. Preheat oven to 350°F.

2. Olive oil should be heated to a medium-high haze in a big skillet.

3. Add diced onion and minced garlic. Cook for 2-3 minutes, until onion is translucent.

4. Add diced sweet potato, cumin, and chili powder. Cook for 5-7 minutes, until sweet potato is tender.

5. Add black beans and 1/2 cup of vegetable broth to the skillet. Stir well.

6. The mixture should thicken after 5 to 7 minutes of simmering.

7. Spread 1/2 cup of salsa on the bottom of a baking dish.

8. The sweet potato and black bean mixture should be stuffed inside each tortilla. The tortillas should be rolled and placed seam-side down in the baking pan.

9. Pour the remaining salsa and vegetable broth over the tortillas.

10. Top with shredded vegan cheese.

11. Bake the dish for 20 to 25 minutes, or until the cheese is bubbling and melted.

12. Serve hot.

Day 3

Breakfast:

Berry Smoothie Bowl

Ingredients:

- 1 cup frozen mixed berries

- 1 banana

- 1/2 cup almond milk

- 1/4 cup rolled oats

- 1 tbsp chia seeds

- Toppings: sliced banana, chopped nuts, fresh berries

Preparation Method:

1. In a blender, combine frozen mixed berries, banana, almond milk, rolled oats, and chia seeds. Blend until smooth.

2. Pour the smoothie into a bowl.

3. Top with sliced banana, chopped nuts, and fresh berries.

4. Serve chilled.

Lunch:

Chickpea Salad

Ingredients:

- 1 can chickpeas, drained and rinsed

- 1 small cucumber, diced

- 1 small red onion, diced

- 1/2 cup cherry tomatoes, halved

- 1/4 cup fresh parsley, chopped

- 2 tbsp lemon juice

- 2 tbsp olive oil

- Salt and pepper, to taste

Preparation Method:

1. In a large bowl, combine chickpeas, diced cucumber, diced red onion, cherry tomatoes, and chopped parsley.

2. Mix the lemon juice, olive oil, salt, and pepper in a small bowl.

3. Mix thoroughly after adding the dressing to the chickpea mixture.

4. Serve cold.

Dinner:

Tofu and Vegetable Stir Fry

Ingredients:

- 1 block firm tofu, diced

- 1 cup mixed vegetables (broccoli, carrots, bell peppers, and snow peas)

- 1 tbsp olive oil

- 2 cloves garlic, minced

- 1 tbsp low-sodium soy sauce

- 1 tsp corn-starch

- Salt and pepper, to taste

Preparation Method:

1. Olive oil should be heated in a big pan over a medium-high heat.

2. Stir for one minute after adding the minced garlic.

3. Mixture of vegetables should be stir-fried for two to three minutes, or until soft.

4. Add diced tofu and stir well.

5. In a small bowl, whisk together soy sauce, corn-starch, and 1/4 cup of water.

6. Pour the sauce over the tofu and vegetables, and stir-fry for an additional 2-3 minutes, until the sauce thickens.

7. Season with salt and pepper.

8. Serve hot.

Day 4

Breakfast:

Vegan Breakfast Burrito

Ingredients:

- 1 small potato, diced

- 1/2 onion, diced

- 1 red bell pepper, diced

- 1/2 cup black beans, drained and rinsed

- 1/2 avocado, diced

- 2 tbsp salsa

- Salt and pepper, to taste

- 1 whole wheat tortilla

Preparation Method:

1. In a skillet, cook the diced potato, onion, and red bell pepper until tender, about 10 minutes.

2. Add black beans and cook for an additional 2-3 minutes.

3. Season with salt and pepper to taste.

4. Warm the whole wheat tortilla in a separate skillet or microwave.

5. Add the potato and bean mixture to the centre of the tortilla.

6. Top with diced avocado and salsa.

7. With the ends tucked in, roll the tortilla up.

8. Serve hot.

Lunch:

Quinoa and Vegetable Bowl

Ingredients:

- 1 cup cooked quinoa

- 1/2 cup roasted sweet potato cubes

- 1/2 cup roasted Brussels sprouts

- 1/2 cup cooked chickpeas

- 1/4 cup sliced almonds

- 2 tbsp lemon juice

- 2 tbsp olive oil

- Salt and pepper, to taste

Preparation Method:

1. In a large bowl, combine cooked quinoa, roasted sweet potato cubes, roasted Brussels sprouts, and cooked chickpeas.

2. Mix the lemon juice, olive oil, salt, and pepper in a small bowl.

3. Mix thoroughly after adding the dressing to the quinoa and veggie mixture.

4. Sprinkle sliced almonds over the top.

5. Serve cold.

Dinner:

Lentil Shepherd's Pie

Ingredients:

- 1 cup green lentils, rinsed and drained

- 1 onion, chopped

- 2 garlic cloves, minced

- 2 medium carrots, diced

- 2 celery stalks, diced

- 1 cup frozen peas

- 1 tsp dried thyme

- 1 tsp dried rosemary

- 2 tbsp tomato paste

- 1 cup vegetable broth

- 2 tbsp olive oil

- Salt and pepper, to taste

- 2 cups mashed potatoes

Preparation Method:

1. Preheat oven to 375°F.

2. Cook the lentils according to package instructions.

3. Olive oil should be heated to a medium-high haze in a big skillet.

4. Add chopped onion and minced garlic and cook for 2-3 minutes, until onion is translucent.

5. Add diced carrots and celery and cook for an additional 5-7 minutes, until vegetables are tender.

6. Add cooked lentils, frozen peas, dried thyme, dried rosemary, tomato paste, and vegetable broth to the skillet.

7. The mixture should thicken after 10 to 15 minutes of simmering.

8. Season with salt and pepper to taste.

9. In a baking dish, evenly distribute the lentil mixture on the bottom.

10. Potato mash should be smeared over the lentil mixture.

11. Bake for 20-25 minutes, until the mashed potatoes are lightly browned.

12. Serve hot.

Day 5

Breakfast:

Overnight Oats

Ingredients:

- 1/2 cup rolled oats

- 1/2 cup almond milk

- 1/2 banana, mashed

- 1/2 tsp vanilla extract

Toppings:

- Fresh berries

- Sliced banana

- Chopped nuts

Preparation Method:

1. In a jar or bowl, combine rolled oats, almond milk, mashed banana, and vanilla extract.

2. Stir well to combine Cover and refrigerate overnight.

3. In the morning, stir the mixture and add desired toppings, such as fresh berries, sliced banana, or chopped nuts.

4. Serve cold.

Lunch:

Vegan Caesar Salad

Ingredients:

- 4 cups chopped Romaine lettuce

- 1/2 cup croutons

- 1/4 cup vegan Caesar dressing (see recipe below)

- 1 tbsp nutritional yeast

- Salt and pepper, to taste

- Vegan Caesar Dressing Ingredients:

- 1/4 cup raw cashews, soaked overnight

- 2 tbsp lemon juice

- 1 tbsp Dijon mustard

- 1 tbsp capers

- 1 garlic clove

- 1/4 cup water

- Salt and pepper, to taste

Preparation Method:

1. In a large bowl, combine chopped Romaine lettuce, croutons, and nutritional yeast.

2. In a blender or food processor, combine soaked cashews, lemon juice, Dijon mustard, capers, garlic clove, water, salt, and pepper.

3. Blend until smooth and creamy.

4. Drizzle the vegan Caesar dressing over the salad and toss well to coat.

5. Serve cold.

Dinner:

Vegan Lentil Chili

Ingredients:

- 1 cup of drained and rinsed green or brown lentils

- 1 onion, chopped

- 2 garlic cloves, minced

- 1 red bell pepper, diced

- 1 green bell pepper, diced

- 1 jalapeno pepper, seeded and diced

- 2 tbsp chili powder

- 1 tbsp ground cumin

- 1 tsp smoked paprika

- 1/4 tsp cayenne pepper (optional)

- 1 can (28 oz) diced tomatoes, undrained

- 1 can (15 oz) washed and drained kidney beans

- 1 can (15 oz) washed and drained black beans

- 2 cups vegetable broth

- 1 tbsp olive oil

- Salt and pepper, to taste

Toppings:

- Diced avocado,

- Chopped cilantro,

- Vegan sour cream (optional)

Preparation Method:

1. Olive oil should be heated in a big pot over a medium-high heat.

2. Add chopped onion, minced garlic, diced red and green bell peppers, and seeded and diced jalapeno pepper.

3. Vegetables should be cooked for 5-7 minutes or until soft.

4. Add chili powder, ground cumin, smoked paprika, and cayenne pepper (if using), and cook for 1-2 minutes, stirring constantly.

5. Add diced tomatoes, drained and rinsed kidney beans and black beans, and vegetable broth to the pot.

6. Bring the mixture to a simmer and add rinsed and drained lentils.

7. Simmer for 25-30 minutes, until lentils are tender and the mixture has thickened.

8. Season with salt and pepper to taste.

9. Serve hot with desired toppings.

Day 6

Breakfast:

Vegan Banana Pancakes

Ingredients:

- 1 cup flour

- 1 tbsp sugar

- 1 tsp baking powder

- 1/4 tsp salt

- 1 ripe banana, mashed

- 1 cup almond milk

- 1 tsp vanilla extract

- 1 tbsp vegetable oil

Preparation Method:

1. Mix the flour, sugar, baking soda, and salt in a big bowl.

2. In a separate bowl, mash the ripe banana and whisk in almond milk, vanilla extract, and vegetable oil.

3. Mix the dry ingredients with the wet components after adding the latter to the former.

4. Heat a non-stick skillet over medium heat and Pour 1/4 cup of batter onto the skillet and cook for 2-3 minutes on each side, until golden brown.

5. Repeat with remaining batter.

6. Serve hot with desired toppings, such as sliced banana, chopped nuts, or maple syrup.

Lunch:

Vegan Buddha Bowl

Ingredients:

- 1 cup quinoa, rinsed and drained

- 1 can (15 oz) washed and drained chickpeas

- 2 cups chopped kale

- 1 avocado, sliced

- 1 carrot, shredded

- 1/4 red onion, sliced

- 1 tbsp olive oil

- 1 tbsp lemon juice

- Salt and pepper, to taste

Preparation Method:

1. Cook quinoa according to package instructions.

2. In a large bowl, combine cooked quinoa, drained and rinsed chickpeas, chopped kale, sliced avocado, shredded carrot, and sliced red onion.

3. Mix the olive oil, lemon juice, salt, and pepper in a small bowl.

4. Drizzle the dressing over the Buddha bowl and toss well to coat.

5. Serve cold or at room temperature.

Dinner:

Vegan Sweet Potato and Black Bean Enchiladas

Ingredients:

- 1 large sweet potato, peeled and diced

- 1 can (15 oz) washed and drained black beans

- 1/2 onion, chopped

- 2 garlic cloves, minced

- 1 tbsp chili powder

- 1 tsp ground cumin

- 1 tsp smoked paprika

- Salt and pepper, to taste

- 1 can (15 oz) enchilada sauce

- 8-10 corn tortillas

- 1/2 cup vegan shredded cheese

Preparation Method:

1. Preheat oven to 375°F.

2. In a large skillet, cook diced sweet potato over medium heat for 5-7 minutes, until tender.

3. Add chopped onion and minced garlic to the skillet and cook for 2-3 minutes, until fragrant.

4. Add drained and rinsed black beans, chili powder, ground cumin, smoked paprika, salt, and pepper to the skillet.

5. Cook for 1-2 minutes, stirring constantly.

6. A 9x13 inch baking dish should contain half of the enchilada sauce.

7. Warm corn tortillas in the microwave for 30 seconds or in a skillet for 10 seconds on each side.

8. Spoon the sweet potato and black bean mixture onto each tortilla and roll tightly.

9. In the baking dish, arrange the rolled tortillas seam-side down.

10. Over the tortillas, spread the leftover enchilada sauce.

11. Top the enchiladas with some vegan cheese shredding.

12. Bake the dish for 20 to 25 minutes, or until heated all the way through and the cheese is melted.

13. Remove foil and bake for an additional 5-10 minutes, until cheese is golden and bubbly.

14. Serve hot with desired toppings, such as sliced avocado, chopped cilantro, or vegan sour cream.

Day 7

Breakfast:

Vegan Breakfast Burrito

Ingredients:

- 1/2 cup black beans, drained and rinsed

- 1/2 cup chopped kale

- 1/4 cup chopped red onion

- 1/4 cup chopped red bell pepper

- 1/4 cup chopped green bell pepper

- 2 tbsp salsa

- Salt and pepper, to taste

- 2 large tortillas

- 1/4 cup vegan shredded cheese

Preparation Method:

1. In a large skillet, cook drained and rinsed black beans over medium heat for 3-4 minutes, until heated through.

2. Add chopped kale, red onion, red bell pepper, and green bell pepper to the skillet and cook for 2-3 minutes, until vegetables are tender.

3. Stir in salsa, salt, and pepper to taste.

4. Warm tortillas in the microwave for 30 seconds or in a skillet for 10 seconds on each side.

5. Spoon the black bean and vegetable mixture onto each tortilla and sprinkle with vegan shredded cheese.

6. Roll the tortillas tightly and serve hot.

Lunch:

Vegan Lentil Soup

Ingredients:

- 1 cup red lentils, rinsed and drained

- 1 onion, chopped

- 2 garlic cloves, minced

- 2 carrots, chopped

- 2 celery stalks, chopped

- 1 tbsp olive oil

- 1 tsp ground cumin

- 1 tsp smoked paprika

- Salt and pepper, to taste

- 4 cups vegetable broth

- 1 can (14 oz) diced tomatoes

- 2 cups chopped kale

Preparation Method:

1. Olive oil is heated over medium heat in a big pot.

2. Add chopped onion and minced garlic to the pot and cook for 2-3 minutes, until fragrant.

3. Add chopped carrots and celery to the pot and cook for 5-7 minutes, until vegetables are tender.

4. Stir in ground cumin, smoked paprika, salt, and pepper to taste.

5. Add rinsed and drained red lentils, vegetable broth, and diced tomatoes to the pot.

6. After bringing the soup to a boil, turn the heat down to low.

7. Cover the pot and simmer for 20-25 minutes, until lentils are tender and soup is heated through.

8. Stir in chopped kale and cook for an additional 5 minutes, until kale is wilted.

9. Serve hot.

Dinner:

Vegan Cauliflower Curry

Ingredients:

- 1 head cauliflower, cut into florets

- 1 onion, chopped

- 2 garlic cloves, minced

- 1 tbsp grated ginger

- 1 can (14 oz) washed and drained chickpeas

- 1 can (14 oz) diced tomatoes

- 1 can (14 oz) coconut milk

- 2 tbsp curry powder

- Salt and pepper, to taste

- Fresh cilantro, chopped, for garnish

Preparation Method:

1. In a large skillet, cook cauliflower florets over medium heat for 5-7 minutes, until slightly tender.

2. Add chopped onion, minced garlic, and grated ginger to the skillet and cook for 2-3 minutes, until fragrant.

3. Stir in drained and rinsed chickpeas, diced tomatoes, coconut milk, curry powder, salt, and pepper to taste.

4. Bring the curry to a simmer and then reduce heat to low.

5. Cover the skillet and cook for 20-25 minutes, until cauliflower is tender and curry is heated through.

6. Serve hot with chopped cilantro as garnish.

These meal ideas should help you create a healthy and satisfying plant-based kidney stone meal plan for 7 days. Remember to also stay hydrated and limit high oxalate foods to prevent kidney stones from forming.

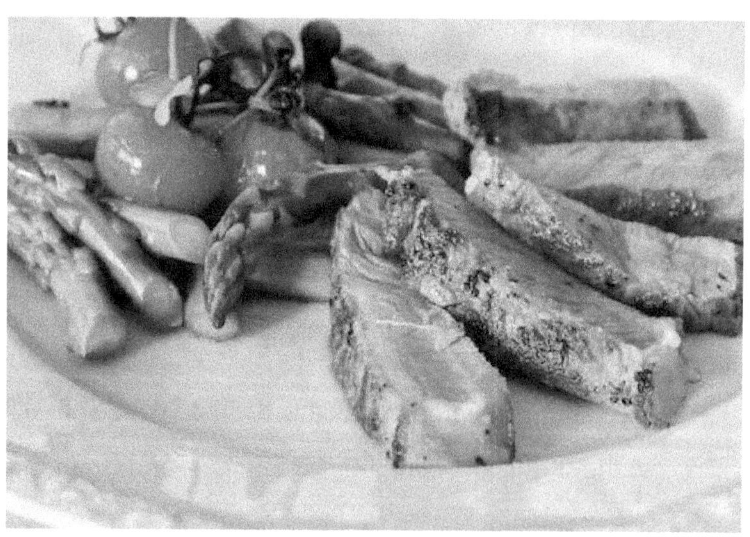

CHAPTER THREE

Plant Based Kidney Stone Recipes

Breakfast

1. Berry Smoothie Bowl

This delicious and nutritious smoothie bowl is packed with antioxidants, fibre, and vitamins to help prevent kidney stones.

Ingredients:

- 1 cup frozen mixed berries

- 1 ripe banana

- 1/2 cup unsweetened almond milk

- 1 tbsp chia seeds

- 1 tbsp honey or maple syrup (optional)

- 1/4 cup granola (optional)

Instructions:

1. Blend the mixed berries, banana, almond milk, chia seeds, and honey/maple syrup in a blender until smooth.

2. Pour the smoothie into a bowl and top with granola, if desired.

3. Serve immediately.

Cooking time: 5 minutes

2. Avocado Toast with Tomato and Basil

This simple and tasty breakfast is high in healthy fats and antioxidants, and low in oxalates (which can contribute to kidney stones).

Ingredients:

- 2 slices whole grain bread

- 1 ripe avocado, mashed

- 1 tomato, sliced

- Fresh basil leaves

- Salt and pepper, to taste

Instructions:

1. Toast the bread until golden brown.

2. Spread the mashed avocado evenly over each slice of toast.

3. Top the avocado with sliced tomato and fresh basil leaves.

4. Season with salt and pepper, to taste.

5. Serve immediately.

Cooking time: 10 minutes

3. Blueberry Oatmeal

This hearty and filling oatmeal is high in fibre and low in oxalates.

Ingredients:

- 1 cup rolled oats

- 2 cups water

- 1/2 cup frozen blueberries

- 1 tbsp chia seeds

- 1/2 tsp vanilla extract

- 1/4 cup chopped walnuts (optional)

Instructions:

1. Combine the oats, water, blueberries, chia seeds, and vanilla extract in a medium saucepan.

2. Bring the mixture to a boil, then reduce the heat to low and simmer for 5-7 minutes, stirring occasionally, until the oatmeal is thick and creamy.

3. Stir in the chopped walnuts, if using.

4. Serve immediately.

Cooking time: 10 minutes

4. Spinach and Mushroom Scramble

This protein-packed scramble is full of healthy greens and mushrooms, which are low in oxalates.

Ingredients:

- 1 cup fresh spinach leaves

- 1 cup sliced mushrooms

- 1/2 cup chopped onion

- 1/2 cup chopped red bell pepper

- 2 tbsp olive oil

- 6 oz firm tofu, crumbled

- Salt and pepper, to taste

Instructions:

1. In a large skillet over medium-high heat, warm the olive oil.

2. Add the onion and red bell pepper and sauté for 2-3 minutes, until softened.

3. Add the mushrooms and spinach and sauté for another 2-3 minutes, until the mushrooms are tender and the spinach is wilted.

4. Add the crumbled tofu and continue to sauté for another 2-3 minutes, until the tofu is heated through and lightly browned.

5. Season with salt and pepper, to taste.

6. Serve immediately.

Cooking time: 15 minutes

5. Quinoa and Fruit Bowl

This protein-packed breakfast bowl is full of fibre and antioxidants to help prevent kidney stones.

Ingredients:

- 1 cup cooked quinoa

- 1 cup mixed fresh fruit (such as berries, chopped apple, and sliced banana)

- 1/4 cup chopped nuts (such as almonds or pecans)

- 1 tbsp honey or maple syrup (optional)

Instructions:

1. In a bowl, combine the cooked quinoa, mixed fresh fruit, and chopped nuts.

2. Drizzle with honey or maple syrup, if desired.

3. Serve immediately.

Cooking time: 15 minutes (for cooking quinoa)

6. Sweet Potato and Black Bean Hash

This savoury and filling hash is loaded with plant-based protein, fibre, and antioxidants.

Ingredients:

- 2 medium sweet potatoes, peeled and diced

- 1 can black beans, drained and rinsed

- 1/2 cup chopped onion

- 1/2 cup chopped red bell pepper

- 2 tbsp olive oil

- 1 tsp smoked paprika

- 1/2 tsp cumin

- Salt and pepper, to taste

Instructions:

1. Over medium-high heat, warm the olive oil in a large skillet.

2. Add the sweet potatoes, onion, and red bell pepper and sauté for 8-10 minutes, until the sweet potatoes are tender and lightly browned.

3. Add the black beans, smoked paprika, cumin, salt, and pepper, and continue to sauté for another 2-3 minutes, until the beans are heated through.

4. Serve immediately.

Cooking time: 20-25 minutes

7. Peanut Butter and Banana Smoothie

This creamy and satisfying smoothie is packed with protein, fibre, and potassium to help prevent kidney stones.

Ingredients:

- 1 ripe banana

- 2 tbsp natural peanut butter

- 1 cup unsweetened almond milk

- 1 tsp honey or maple syrup (optional)

- 1/2 cup ice cubes

Instructions:

1. Blend the banana, peanut butter, almond milk, honey/maple syrup (if using), and ice cubes in a blender until smooth.

2. Serve immediately.

Cooking time: 5 minutes

8. Tofu Breakfast Burrito

This protein-packed breakfast burrito is a tasty and satisfying way to start the day.

Ingredients:

- 1/2 block firm tofu, crumbled

- 1/2 cup chopped onion

- 1/2 cup chopped red bell pepper

- 2 tbsp olive oil

- 1/2 tsp cumin

- Salt and pepper, to taste

- 1 whole grain tortilla

- 1/4 cup salsa (optional)

Instructions:

1. Large skillet set over medium-high heat to warm the olive oil.

2. Add the onion and red bell pepper and sauté for 2-3 minutes, until softened.

3. Add the crumbled tofu, cumin, salt, and pepper, and continue to sauté for another 2-3 minutes, until the tofu is heated through and lightly browned.

4. Warm the tortilla in the microwave or on a skillet for a few seconds.

5. Spoon the tofu mixture onto the tortilla and top with salsa, if desired.

6. Fold the tortilla over the filling to create a burrito.

7. Serve immediately.

Cooking time: 15 minutes

9. Oats overnighted with berries and chia seeds

This easy and nutritious breakfast can be made the night before for a quick and healthy grab-and-go option.

Ingredients:

- 1 cup rolled oats

- 1 cup unsweetened almond milk

- 1 tbsp chia seeds

- 1/2 cup frozen mixed berries

- 1 tbsp honey or maple syrup (optional)

Instructions:

1. Combine the oats, almond milk, chia seeds, frozen berries, and honey/maple syrup (if using) in a jar or container with a lid.

2. Stir well to combine.

3. Cover the jar/container and refrigerate overnight.

4. In the morning, give the mixture a good stir and add more almond milk, if needed, to achieve your desired consistency.

5. Serve chilled.

Cooking time: 5 minutes (plus overnight refrigeration)

10. Vegan Breakfast Tacos

These tasty breakfast tacos are loaded with plant-based protein, fibre, and flavour.

Ingredients:

- 1/2 block firm tofu, crumbled

- 1/2 cup black beans, drained and rinsed

- 1/2 cup chopped onion

- 1/2 cup chopped red bell pepper

- 2 tbsp olive oil

- 1/2 tsp cumin

- Salt and pepper, to taste

- 4 small corn tortillas

- 1/4 cup salsa (optional)

Instructions:

1. In a large skillet over medium-high heat, warm the olive oil.

2. Add the onion and red bell pepper and sauté for 2-3 minutes, until softened.

3. Add the crumbled tofu, black beans, cumin, salt, and pepper, and continue to sauté for another 2-3 minutes, until the tofu is heated through and lightly browned.

4. Warm the tortillas in the microwave or on a skillet for a few seconds.

5. Spoon the tofu mixture onto the tortillas and top with salsa, if desired.

6. Serve immediately.

Cooking time: 15 minutes

These 10 plant-based breakfast recipes are not only delicious, but also packed with nutrients that can help prevent kidney stones.

Give them a try and start your day on a healthy note!

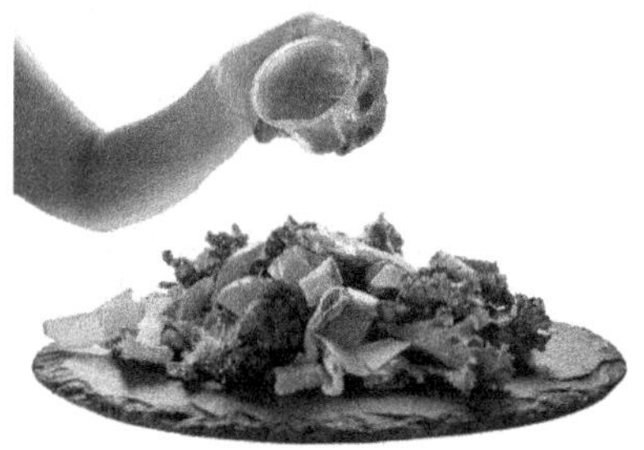

CHAPTER FOUR

Lunch

1. Quinoa Salad with Avocado Dressing

This refreshing quinoa salad is loaded with nutrients and flavour. The creamy avocado dressing is a delicious addition that will make this dish a hit with everyone.

Ingredients:

- 1 cup quinoa

- 2 cups water

- 1 can chickpeas, drained and rinsed

- 1 red bell pepper, diced

- 1/2 red onion, diced

- 1 avocado

- 1/4 cup olive oil

- 1/4 cup lime juice

- 1 clove garlic

- Salt and pepper to taste

Instructions:

1. After thoroughly cleaning it, put the quinoa and water to a pot. When the quinoa is ready, simmer for 15 to 20 minutes after bringing to a boil.

2. In a large bowl, combine the chickpeas, bell pepper, and red onion.

3. In a blender or food processor, combine the avocado, olive oil, lime juice, garlic, salt, and pepper. Blend until smooth.

4. Add the cooked quinoa to the bowl with the chickpeas and vegetables. Pour the avocado dressing over the top and toss to combine.

5. Serve right away or keep chilled for up to three days.

Cooking time: 25 minutes

2. Lentil Soup with Spinach

This hearty lentil soup is packed with fibre and protein, making it a filling and satisfying meal. The addition of spinach adds a pop of colour and nutrients.

Ingredients:

- 1 cup brown lentils

- 6 cups vegetable broth

- 1 onion, diced

- 2 cloves garlic, minced

- 2 carrots, diced

- 2 stalks celery, diced

- 1 teaspoon dried thyme

- 1/2 teaspoon dried oregano

- 1/2 teaspoon paprika

- 1 bay leaf

- 2 cups fresh spinach

- Salt and pepper to taste

Instructions:

1. Rinse the lentils and add them to a large pot with the vegetable broth, onion, garlic, carrots, celery, thyme, oregano, paprika, and bay leaf.

2. The mixture should be brought to a boil before being simmered for 30 to 40 minutes, depending on how tender you like your lentils.

3. Remove the bay leaf and stir in the spinach until wilted.

4. Season with salt and pepper to taste.

5. Serve hot with crusty bread.

Cooking time: 45 minutes

3. Sweet Potato and Black Bean Chili

This hearty chili is packed with flavour and nutrients. The sweet potatoes add a touch of sweetness, while the black beans provide protein and fibre.

Ingredients:

- 2 sweet potatoes, peeled and diced

* 1 onion, diced

* 2 cloves garlic, minced

* 1 red bell pepper, diced

* 1 can diced tomatoes

* 1 can black beans, drained and rinsed

* 1 tablespoon chili powder

* 1 teaspoon ground cumin

* Salt and pepper to taste

Instructions:

1. Heat a large pot over medium-high heat. Add the sweet potatoes, onion, garlic, and red bell pepper. Cook the vegetables for 5-7 minutes, or until they are tender.

2. Add the diced tomatoes (with their juice), black beans, chili powder, cumin, salt, and pepper. Stir to combine.

3. Bring the mixture to a boil, then reduce the heat and simmer for 20-25 minutes or until the sweet potatoes are tender.

4. Lentil and Vegetable Stir-Fry

This colourful and flavourful stir-fry is packed with veggies and protein-rich lentils. It's a quick and easy lunch option that will keep you satisfied for hours.

Ingredients:

- 1 cup cooked lentils

- 2 cups mixed vegetables (such as bell pepper, broccoli, zucchini, and carrots), sliced

- 1 onion, sliced

- 2 cloves garlic, minced

- 1 tablespoon soy sauce

- 1 tablespoon sesame oil

- Salt and pepper to taste

Instructions:

1. Heat a large skillet over medium-high heat. Add the mixed vegetables, onion, and garlic. Cook the vegetables for 5-7 minutes, or until they are crisp-tender.

2. Add the cooked lentils, soy sauce, sesame oil, salt, and pepper. Stir to combine and cook for an additional 2-3 minutes or until the lentils are heated through.

3. Serve hot over brown rice or quinoa.

Cooking time: 15-20 minutes

5. Vegan Caesar Salad

This vegan Caesar salad is a healthier twist on the classic dish. It's packed with flavour and nutrients, and the creamy dressing is made with heart-healthy cashews.

Ingredients:

For the dressing:

- soaking for at least two hours, one cup of cashews

- 1/4 cup lemon juice

- 2 cloves garlic

- 1/4 cup nutritional yeast

- 1 tablespoon Dijon mustard

- 1/4 cup water

- Salt and pepper to taste

For the salad:

- 1 head romaine lettuce, chopped

- 1/2 cup croutons

- 1/4 cup vegan parmesan cheese (optional)

Instructions:

1. To make the dressing, drain and rinse the soaked cashews. Add them to a blender with the lemon juice, garlic, nutritional yeast, Dijon mustard, water, salt, and pepper. Blend until smooth and creamy.

2. In a large bowl, combine the chopped romaine lettuce, croutons, and vegan parmesan cheese (if using).

3. Drizzle the Caesar dressing over the top and toss to combine.

4. Serve immediately.

Cooking time: 10 minutes (plus soaking time)

6. Vegan Lentil Sloppy Joes

These vegan lentil sloppy joes are a healthier take on the classic sandwich. They're packed with fibre and protein, and the tangy tomato sauce is sure to satisfy your cravings.

Ingredients:

- 1 cup brown lentils

- 2 cups vegetable broth

- 1 onion, diced

- 2 cloves garlic, minced

- 1 red bell pepper, diced

- 1 can tomato sauce

- 2 tablespoons maple syrup

- 1 tablespoon apple cider vinegar

- 1 tablespoon chili powder

- Salt and pepper to taste

- Hamburger buns or whole-grain bread

Instructions:

1. Rinse the lentils and add them to a large pot with the vegetable broth, onion, garlic, and red bell pepper.

2. The mixture should be brought to a boil before being simmered for 30 to 40 minutes, depending on how tender you like your lentils.

3. Stir in the tomato sauce, maple syrup, apple cider vinegar, chili powder, salt, and pepper. Simmer the sauce for a further 10 to 15 minutes, or until it has thickened.

4. Serve the lentil mixture on hamburger buns or whole-grain bread.

Cooking time: 45-50 minutes

7. Greek Salad with Quinoa

This Greek salad with quinoa is a light and refreshing lunch option. It's packed with vegetables and protein-rich quinoa, and the tangy dressing adds a burst of flavour.

Ingredients:

For the dressing:

- 1/4 cup olive oil

- 2 tablespoons red wine vinegar

- 1 tablespoon lemon juice

- 1 teaspoon dried oregano

- Salt and pepper to taste

For the salad:

- 1 cup cooked quinoa

- 1 cucumber, diced

- 1 tomato, diced

- 1/2 red onion, sliced

- 1/2 cup Kalamata olives

- 1/2 cup crumbled feta cheese (optional)

Instructions:

1. To make the dressing, whisk together the olive oil, red wine vinegar, lemon juice, oregano, salt, and pepper in a small bowl.

2. In a large bowl, combine the cooked quinoa, cucumber, tomato, red onion, Kalamata olives, and feta cheese (if using).

3. Over the top, drizzle the dressing and toss to incorporate.

4. Offer cold.

Cooking time: 20-25 minutes

8. Spicy Vegan Chili

This spicy vegan chili is packed with flavour and plant-based protein. It's a great option for a filling and satisfying lunch that will keep you going all day.

Ingredients:

- 1 tablespoon olive oil

- 1 onion, diced

- 2 cloves garlic, minced

- 1 red bell pepper, diced

- 1 jalapeno pepper, diced

- 1 can diced tomatoes

- 1 can kidney beans, drained and rinsed

- 1 can black beans, drained and rinsed

- 1 tablespoon chili powder

- 1 teaspoon ground cumin

- Salt and pepper to taste

Optional toppings:

- Avocado

- Cilantro

- Vegan sour cream

Instructions:

1. Heat the olive oil on a high heat in a big saucepan. Add the red bell pepper, jalapeño pepper, onion, and garlic. Cook the vegetables for 5-7 minutes, or until they are soft.

2. The diced tomatoes, kidney beans, black beans, cumin, chili powder, salt, and pepper should all be added. To blend, stir.

3. Bring the mixture to a boil, then reduce the heat and simmer for 20-25 minutes or until the chili has thickened.

4. Serve hot with avocado, cilantro, and vegan sour cream (if desired).

Cooking time: 30-35 minutes

9. Vegan Falafel Wrap

This vegan falafel wrap is a delicious and satisfying lunch option. It's packed with protein and fibre, and the creamy tahini sauce adds a flavourful kick.

Ingredients:

For the falafel:

- 1 can chickpeas, drained and rinsed

- 1/2 onion, chopped

- 2 cloves garlic, minced

- 1/4 cup chopped fresh parsley

- 1 tablespoon ground cumin

- 1 tablespoon ground coriander

- Salt and pepper to taste

- 1/4 cup chickpea flour

- 2 tablespoons olive oil

For the tahini sauce:

- 1/4 cup tahini

- 2 tablespoons lemon juice

- 1 clove garlic, minced

- Salt and pepper to taste

- Water, as needed

For the wrap:

- Whole-grain tortillas

- Shredded lettuce

- Diced tomato

- Diced cucumber

- Sliced red onion

Instructions:

1. To make the falafel, add the chickpeas, onion, garlic, parsley, cumin, coriander, salt, and pepper to a food processor. The mixture should be mixed but slightly lumpy after a few pulses.

2. Stir in the chickpea flour until the mixture is well-combined.

3. In a large skillet over medium-high heat, warm the olive oil. Form the chickpea mixture into small balls and flatten them slightly. Place them in the skillet and cook for 2-3 minutes on each side, or until golden brown.

4. To make the tahini sauce, whisk together the tahini, lemon juice, garlic, salt, and pepper in a small bowl. To thin the sauce to the desired consistency, add water as necessary.

5. To assemble the wraps, spread a generous amount of tahini sauce on a tortilla. Top with shredded lettuce, diced tomato, diced cucumber, sliced red onion, and a few falafel patties. The tortilla should be securely rolled, with the ends tucked in as you go.

6. Serve immediately.

Cooking time: 30-35 minutes

10. Lentil and Vegetable Stir-Fry

This lentil and vegetable stir-fry is a healthy and delicious lunch option that's packed with protein and fibre. The mix of colourful vegetables adds a variety of vitamins and minerals, and the stir-fry sauce brings everything together with a burst of flavour.

Ingredients:

For the stir-fry sauce:

- 1/4 cup low-sodium soy sauce

- 1/4 cup vegetable broth

- 1 tablespoon corn-starch

- 1 tablespoon honey

- 1 tablespoon rice vinegar

- 1 teaspoon grated ginger

- 1 garlic clove, minced

For the stir-fry:

- 1 tablespoon olive oil

- 1 onion, chopped

- 2 cloves garlic, minced

- 1 red bell pepper, sliced

- 1 zucchini, sliced

- 1 cup cooked lentils

- 2 cups cooked brown rice

Instructions:

1. To make the stir-fry sauce, whisk together the soy sauce, vegetable broth, corn-starch, honey, rice vinegar, ginger, and garlic in a small bowl.

2. In a sizable skillet or wok set over medium-high heat, warm the olive oil. Add the onion and garlic and cook for 2-3 minutes or until the vegetables are tender.

3. Add the red bell pepper and zucchini to the skillet and cook for another 2-3 minutes or until the vegetables are crisp-tender.

4. Add the cooked lentils and stir-fry sauce to the skillet. Cook for 2-3 minutes or until the sauce has thickened and the lentils are heated through.

5. Serve the stir-fry over a bed of cooked brown rice.

Cooking time: 25-30 minutes.

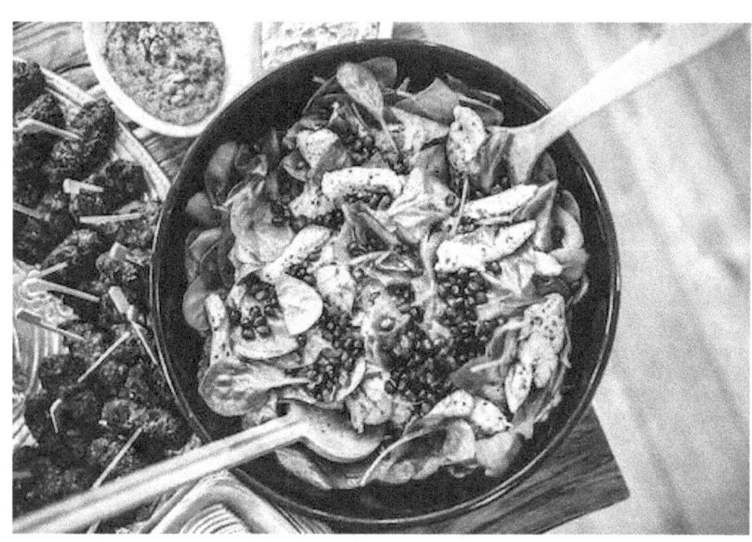

CHAPTER FIVE

Dinner

1. Lentil and Vegetable Stir Fry

This stir fry recipe is packed with kidney stone fighting ingredients such as lentils, vegetables, and spices.

Ingredients:

- 1 cup lentils

- 2 cups mixed vegetables (e.g., broccoli, carrots, bell peppers, snow peas)

- 1 onion, chopped

- 2 cloves garlic, minced

- 1 tsp ginger, grated

- 2 tbsp soy sauce

- 1 tbsp corn-starch

- 1 tsp sesame oil

- Salt and pepper to taste

Instructions:

1. Cook the lentils according to package instructions.

2. In a large pan or wok, sauté the onion, garlic, and ginger until fragrant.

3. When the vegetables are soft, add the mixed vegetables.

4. Mix together the soy sauce, corn-starch, and sesame oil, then add to the pan and cook for a few more minutes.

5. Serve the stir fry over the cooked lentils.

Cooking time: 30 minutes

2. Sweet Potato and Black Bean Enchiladas

These enchiladas are filled with black beans and sweet potatoes, both of which are great for preventing kidney stones.

Ingredients:

- 6 whole wheat tortillas

- 2 sweet potatoes, diced

- 1 can black beans, drained and rinsed

- 1 onion, chopped

- 2 cloves garlic, minced

- 1 tsp cumin

- 1 tsp chili powder

- 1/2 cup tomato sauce

- 1/2 cup vegetable broth

- Salt and pepper to taste

Instructions:

1. Preheat the oven to 350°F.

2. The onion and garlic should be sautéed until aromatic in a big pan.

3. Add the sweet potatoes, black beans, cumin, chili powder, tomato sauce, and vegetable broth to the pan.

4. Cook until the sweet potatoes are tender.

5. Roll up the tortillas after dividing the filling between them.

6. Bake the enchiladas for 15-20 minutes in a baking dish.

7. Serve with avocado and salsa.

Cooking time: 45 minutes

3. Quinoa and Chickpea Salad

This salad is a great way to get in a variety of kidney stone preventing ingredients, including quinoa, chickpeas, and leafy greens.

Ingredients:

- 1 cup quinoa

- 1 can chickpeas, drained and rinsed

- 2 cups mixed greens

- 1 red bell pepper, diced

- 1/4 cup chopped fresh parsley

- 1/4 cup chopped fresh mint

- 1/4 cup olive oil

- 2 tbsp lemon juice

- Salt and pepper to taste

Instructions:

1. Cook the quinoa according to package instructions.

2. In a large bowl, mix together the cooked quinoa, chickpeas, mixed greens, red bell pepper, parsley, and mint.

3. Mix the olive oil, lemon juice, salt, and pepper in another bowl.

4. After adding the dressing, toss the salad to incorporate.

Cooking time: 20 minutes

4. Broccoli and Tofu Stir Fry

This stir fry is a great way to get in some calcium, which can help prevent kidney stones.

Ingredients:

- 1 block tofu, cubed

- 2 cups broccoli florets

- 1 red bell pepper, sliced

- 1 onion, sliced

- 2 cloves garlic, minced

- 1 tsp ginger, grated

- 2 tbsp soy sauce

- 1 tbsp corn-starch

- 1 tsp sesame oil

- Salt and pepper to taste

Instructions:

1. In a large pan or wok, sauté the tofu until browned on all sides.

2. Add the broccoli, red bell pepper, onion, garlic, and ginger to the pan and cook until tender.

3. Mix together the soy sauce, corn-starch, and sesame oil, then add to the pan and cook for a few more minutes.

4. Serve the stir fry over quinoa or brown rice.

Cooking time: 30 minutes

5. Spinach and Mushroom Risotto

This creamy risotto is filled with spinach and mushrooms, which are great for preventing kidney stones.

Ingredients:

- 1 cup arborio rice

- 4 cups vegetable broth

- 1 onion, chopped

- 2 cloves garlic, minced

- 1 cup sliced mushrooms

- 2 cups packed fresh spinach

- 1/4 cup nutritional yeast

- 2 tbsp olive oil

- Salt and pepper to taste

Instructions:

1. Olive oil should be heated in a sizable pot over medium heat.

2. Once aromatic, add the onion and garlic.

3. Stir the arborio rice into the oil after adding it.

4. Slowly add the vegetable broth, 1/2 cup at a time, stirring constantly until the broth is absorbed.

5. Add the mushrooms and spinach and continue to cook until the rice is tender.

6. Salt and pepper to taste, then stir in the nutritional yeast.

Cooking time: 45 minutes

6. Roasted Vegetable Quinoa Bowl

This quinoa bowl is filled with roasted vegetables and quinoa, both of which are great for preventing kidney stones.

Ingredients:

- 1 cup quinoa

- 2 cups mixed vegetables (e.g., sweet potato, zucchini, bell peppers)

- 1 onion, chopped

- 2 cloves garlic, minced

- 1 tsp cumin

- 1 tsp chili powder

- 2 tbsp olive oil

- Salt and pepper to taste

Instructions:

1. Preheat the oven to 400°F.

2. Cook the quinoa according to package instructions.

3. In a large bowl, toss the mixed vegetables with the onion, garlic, cumin, chili powder, olive oil, salt, and pepper.

4. Spread the vegetables out on a baking sheet and roast for 20-25 minutes, or until tender and browned.

5. Serve the vegetables over the cooked quinoa.

Cooking time: 40 minutes

7. Cauliflower Rice Stir Fry

This stir fry is made with cauliflower rice instead of traditional rice, making it a great low-carb option that is still packed with kidney stone preventing ingredients.

Ingredients:

- 1 head cauliflower, riced

- 2 cups mixed vegetables (e.g., carrots, bell peppers, snow peas)

- 1 onion, chopped

- 2 cloves garlic, minced

- 1 tsp ginger, grated

- 2 tbsp soy sauce

- 1 tbsp corn-starch

- 1 tsp sesame oil

- Salt and pepper to taste

Instructions:

1. In a large pan or wok, sauté the onion, garlic, and ginger until fragrant.

2. When the vegetables are soft, add the mixed vegetables.

3. Add the cauliflower rice to the pan and cook until tender.

4. Mix together the soy sauce, corn-starch, and sesame oil, then add to the pan and cook for a few more minutes.

5. Serve the stir fry topped with chopped green onions and sesame seeds.

Cooking time: 30 minutes

8. Chickpea and Sweet Potato Curry

This curry is packed with kidney stone preventing ingredients like chickpeas, sweet potatoes, and spinach.

Ingredients:

- 1 can chickpeas, drained and rinsed

- 2 sweet potatoes, peeled and cubed

- 1 onion, chopped

- 2 cloves garlic, minced

- 1 tbsp curry powder

- 1 can diced tomatoes

- 1 cup vegetable broth

- 2 cups packed fresh spinach

- 2 tbsp olive oil

- Salt and pepper to taste

Instructions:

1. Olive oil should be heated in a sizable pot over medium heat.

2. Once aromatic, add the onion and garlic.

3. Add the curry powder and cook for a few more minutes.

4. Add the chickpeas, sweet potatoes, diced tomatoes, and vegetable broth to the pot and bring to a simmer.

5. Until the sweet potatoes are cooked through, simmer for 20 to 25 minutes.

6. Add the spinach and stir until it wilts.

7. Season with salt and pepper to taste.

Cooking time: 45 minutes

9. Lentil Shepherd's Pie

This hearty and comforting shepherd's pie is made with lentils, which are great for preventing kidney stones.

Ingredients:

- 2 cups cooked lentils

- 2 cups mixed vegetables (e.g., carrots, peas, corn)

- 1 onion, chopped

- 2 cloves garlic, minced

- 1 tbsp tomato paste

- 1 tbsp flour

- 1 cup vegetable broth

- 2 tbsp olive oil

- Salt and pepper to taste

- 3 cups mashed potatoes

Instructions:

1. Preheat the oven to 350°F.

2. Olive oil should be heated in a sizable pot over medium heat.

3. Once aromatic, add the onion and garlic.

4. When the vegetables are soft, add the mixed vegetables.

5. Add the cooked lentils, tomato paste, flour, and vegetable broth to the pot and bring to a simmer.

6. Simmer the mixture for 10 to 15 minutes, or until it has thickened.

7. Season with salt and pepper to taste.

8. Spread the lentil mixture into a large baking dish.

9. Spread the mashed potatoes equally over the lentil mixture before adding the topping.

10. Bake for 25-30 minutes, or until the potatoes are browned and the filling is heated through.

Cooking time: 1 hour

10. Broiled Portobello Mushrooms with Roasted Vegetables

This simple yet delicious dish features portobello mushrooms, which are high in potassium and great for preventing kidney stones.

Ingredients:

- 4 large portobello mushrooms

- 2 cups mixed vegetables (e.g., carrots, broccoli, bell peppers)

- 1 onion, chopped

- 2 cloves garlic, minced

- 2 tbsp balsamic vinegar

- 2 tbsp olive oil

- Salt and pepper to taste

Instructions:

1. Preheat the broiler.

2. In a large bowl, toss the mixed vegetables with the onion, garlic, balsamic vinegar, olive oil, salt, and pepper.

3. Spread the vegetables out on a baking sheet and broil for 5-7 minutes, or until tender and browned.

4. Meanwhile, clean the portobello mushrooms and remove the stems.

5. Place the mushrooms on a broiler pan, gill side up.

6. Broil the mushrooms for 5-7 minutes, or until tender and juicy.

7. Serve the mushrooms topped with the roasted vegetables.

Cooking time: 20 minutes

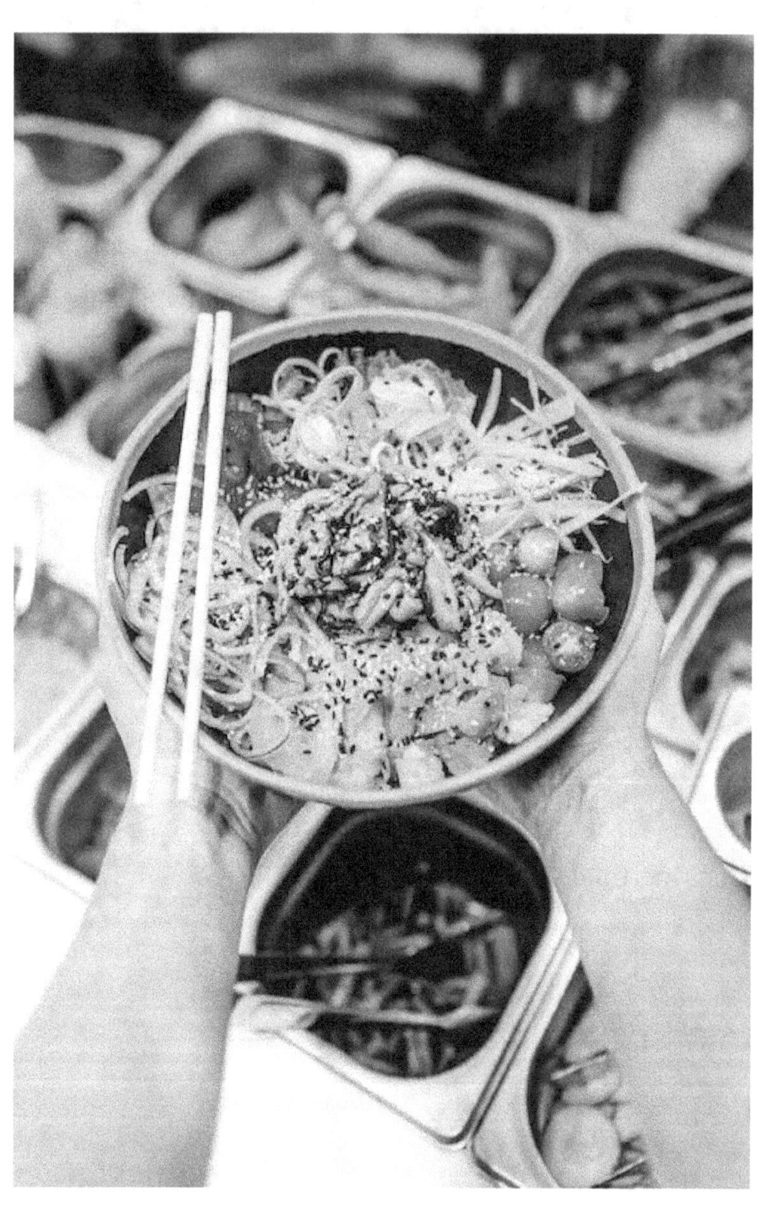

CHAPTER SIX

Dessert

1. Chocolate Chia Pudding

Ingredients:

- 1/4 cup chia seeds

- 1 cup almond milk

- 2 tbsp cocoa powder

- 2 tbsp maple syrup

- 1/2 tsp vanilla extract

- Pinch of salt

Instructions:

1. In a medium bowl, whisk together chia seeds, almond milk, cocoa powder, maple syrup, vanilla extract, and salt.

2. Once the pudding has thickened, cover it and place it in the refrigerator for at least two hours or overnight.

3. Serve chilled, topped with fresh berries, if desired.

Cooking Time: 2 hours minimum

2. Blueberry Oat Bars

Ingredients:

- 2 cups rolled oats

- 1/2 cup almond flour

- 1/4 cup coconut oil, melted

- 1/4 cup maple syrup

- 1 tsp vanilla extract

- 1/2 tsp baking powder

- 1/4 tsp salt

- 1 cup blueberries

Instructions:

1. Preheat oven to 350°F (175°C) and line a 9x9 inch baking dish with parchment paper.

2. In a large bowl, combine oats, almond flour, melted coconut oil, maple syrup, vanilla extract, baking powder, and salt.

3. Mix until well combined and crumbly.

4. In the bottom of the baking dish that has been prepared, press half of the oat mixture evenly.

5. Sprinkle the blueberries over the oat mixture.

6. Crumble the remaining oat mixture over the blueberries.

7. Bake for 30-35 minutes, or until golden brown around the edges.

8. Let cool before slicing into bars.

Cooking Time: 35 minutes

3. Strawberry Banana Nice Cream

Ingredients:

- 2 frozen bananas

- 1 cup frozen strawberries

- 1/4 cup almond milk

- 1 tsp vanilla extract

Instructions:

1. Add the frozen bananas, frozen strawberries, almond milk, and vanilla extract to a high-speed blender or food processor.

2. Blend until smooth and creamy.

3. Serve immediately, garnished with fresh berries, if desired.

Cooking Time: None

4. Almond Flour Chocolate Chip Cookies

Ingredients:

- 2 cups almond flour

- 1/2 cup coconut sugar

- 1/2 tsp baking powder

- 1/2 tsp baking soda

- Pinch of salt

- 1/4 cup coconut oil, melted

- 1 flax egg (made from 1 tbsp. powdered flaxseed and 3 tbsp. water)

- 1 tsp vanilla extract

- 1/2 cup dark chocolate chips

Instructions:

1. Set a baking sheet on the counter and preheat the oven to 350°F (175°C).

2. In a large bowl, whisk together almond flour, coconut sugar, baking powder, baking soda, and salt.

3. In a separate bowl, whisk together melted coconut oil, flax egg, and vanilla extract.

4. Stir to thoroughly incorporate the dry ingredients before adding the wet ingredients.

5. Fold in the dark chocolate chips.

6. Scoop dough onto the preheated baking sheet in tablespoon-sized chunks.

7. Bake for 10 to 12 minutes, or until golden brown around the edges.

8. Allow to cool for five minutes on the baking sheet before transferring to a wire rack to finish cooling.

Cooking Time: 12 minutes

5. Banana Bread Bites

Ingredients:

- 2 ripe bananas, mashed

- 1/4 cup almond butter

- 1/4 cup maple syrup

- 1 tsp vanilla extract

- 1 1/2 cups rolled oats

- 1 tsp baking powder

- 1/2 tsp cinnamon

- Pinch of salt

Instructions:

1. Set a baking sheet on the counter and preheat the oven to 350°F (175°C).

2. In a large bowl, mix together mashed bananas, almond butter, maple syrup, and vanilla extract.

3. In a separate bowl, mix together rolled oats, baking powder, cinnamon, and salt.

4. The dry components should be mixed thoroughly with the wet ingredients after being added.

5. Use a cookie scoop or spoon to drop tablespoon-sized portions of the dough onto the prepared baking sheet.

6. Until golden brown, bake for 12 to 15 minutes.

7. Allow to cool for five minutes on the baking sheet before transferring to a wire rack to finish cooling.

Cooking Time: 15 minutes

Snack

1. Roasted Chickpeas

Ingredients:

- 1 can of chickpeas, drained and rinsed

- 1 tsp olive oil

- 1 tsp paprika

- 1 tsp garlic powder

- 1 tsp onion powder

- Salt and pepper to taste

Instructions:

1. Preheat the oven to 400°F (200°C).

2. With a paper towel, dry the chickpeas off.

3. In a bowl, mix the olive oil, paprika, garlic powder, onion powder, salt, and pepper.

4. Mix thoroughly after adding the chickpeas to the bowl.

5. On a baking sheet covered with parchment paper, spread the chickpeas out.

6. Roast in the oven for 20-25 minutes or until crispy, stirring halfway through.

7. Let cool and enjoy.

Cooking Time: 25 minutes

2. Cucumber and Hummus Bites

Ingredients:

- 1 cucumber

- 1/2 cup hummus

- 1 tbsp chopped parsley

Instructions:

1. Cut the cucumber into thin slices.

2. Spread a dollop of hummus on each cucumber slice.

3. Sprinkle chopped parsley on top.

4. Serve and enjoy.

Cooking Time: 10 minutes

3. Vegan Protein Balls

Ingredients:

- 1 cup dates, pitted

- 1/2 cup almonds

- 1/4 cup chia seeds

- 1/4 cup hemp seeds

- 1/4 cup cocoa powder

- 1/4 cup unsweetened shredded coconut

- 1/4 tsp sea salt

- 1-2 tbsp water (as needed)

Instructions:

1. Add the dates, almonds, chia seeds, hemp seeds, cocoa powder, shredded coconut, and sea salt to a food processor.

2. Pulse until everything is well combined and a dough forms.

3. To reach the desired consistency, add water as necessary.

4. On a baking sheet lined with paper, form the dough into balls.

5. Refrigerate until hard, or for at least 30 minutes.

6. Serve and enjoy.

Cooking Time: 40 minutes

4. Sweet Potato Chips

Ingredients:

- 2 sweet potatoes

- 2 tbsp olive oil

- 1/2 tsp sea salt

- 1/2 tsp smoked paprika

- 1/2 tsp garlic powder

Instructions:

1. Preheat the oven to 375°F (190°C).

2. Wash the sweet potatoes and slice them into thin rounds.

3. In a bowl, mix the olive oil, sea salt, smoked paprika, and garlic powder.

4. Add the sweet potato slices to the bowl and mix well.

5. On a baking sheet covered with parchment paper, distribute the sweet potato slices.

6. Bake in the oven for 15-20 minutes or until crispy, flipping halfway through.

7. Let cool and enjoy.

Cooking Time: 25 minutes

5. Zucchini Fritters

Ingredients:

- 2 medium zucchinis

- 1/4 cup chickpea flour

- 1/4 cup nutritional yeast

- 1/4 tsp garlic powder

- 1/4 tsp onion powder

- 1/4 tsp sea salt

- 1/4 tsp black pepper

- 2 tbsp olive oil

Instructions:

1. Utilize a box grater or food processor to grate the zucchini.

2. Sea salt should be added to the grated zucchini before placing it in a colander over a basin.

3. Let the zucchini sit for 10-15 minutes to release excess water.

4. Use a clean towel or paper towels to squeeze out any remaining water from the zucchini.

5. In a bowl, mix the zucchini, chickpea flour, nutritional yeast, garlic powder, onion powder, sea salt, and black pepper.

6. Over medium heat, warm the olive oil in a skillet.

7. Scoop 1/4 cup of the zucchini mixture into the skillet for each fritter.

8. Flatten the mixture into a pancake shape and cook for 3-4 minutes on each side or until golden brown.

9. Repeat with the remaining mixture.

10. Serve and enjoy.

Cooking Time: 30 minutes

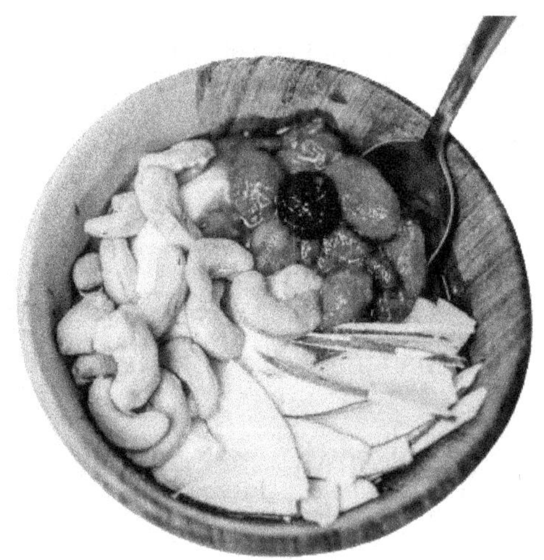

CONCLUSION

In conclusion, a plant-based kidney stone cookbook can be an excellent resource for individuals looking to prevent or manage kidney stones.

By incorporating a variety of nutrient-dense, plant-based foods, individuals can optimize their diet to support healthy kidney function.

The recipes in a plant-based kidney stone cookbook are designed to be both delicious and nutritious, making it easy for individuals to transition to a more plant-focused diet.

Ingredients such as whole grains, legumes, fruits, and vegetables provide a variety of vitamins, minerals, and antioxidants that can help to prevent the formation of kidney stones.

In addition to providing recipes, a plant-based kidney stone cookbook may also offer guidance on dietary modifications that can help to reduce the risk of kidney stone formation. This may include information on limiting high-oxalate foods, such as spinach, rhubarb, and beets, and increasing intake of calcium-rich foods, such as tofu, broccoli, and kale.

Overall, a plant-based kidney stone cookbook can be an invaluable resource for individuals looking to make dietary changes to support kidney health. By incorporating a variety of plant-based foods into their diet, individuals can reduce their risk of kidney stone formation while also improving their overall health and wellbeing.

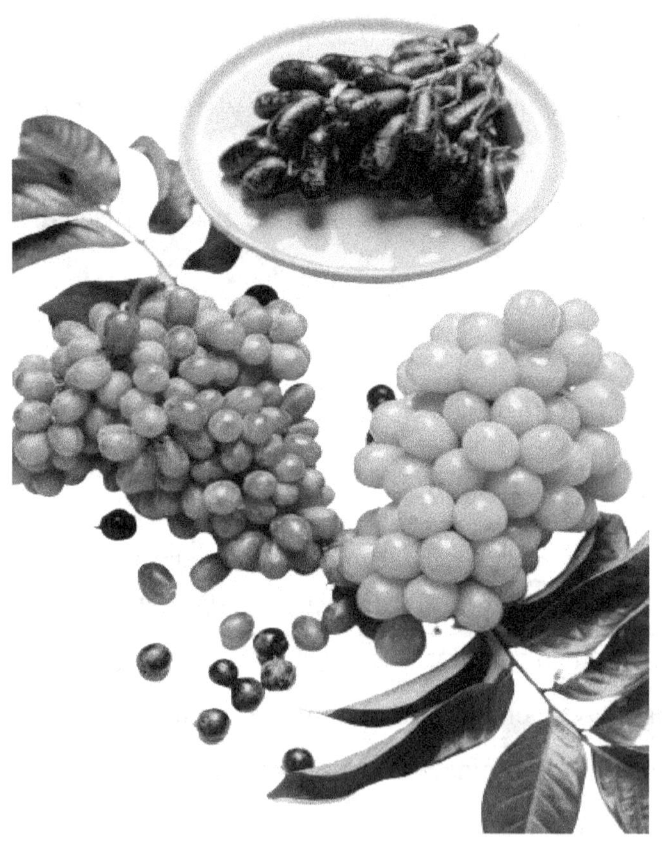

www.ingramcontent.com/pod-product-compliance
Lightning Source LLC
Chambersburg PA
CBHW070951250726

48663CB00002B/169

* 9 7 9 8 8 5 4 6 9 6 8 3 8 *